Table of Contents

LYMPHEDEMA DIET

Lymph is a protein rich fluid found in the lymphatic system. It contains white blood cells which help remove waste and play a key role in our immunity. If lymph fluid accumulates for some reason, it can cause abnormal swelling in the extremities, abdomen, face or neck.

LYMPHEDEMA DIET RECIPES

1. Mango Overnight Oats

Prep Time: 10 mins

Total Time: 3 hrs 10 mins

Servings: 1

Ingredients

- ½ cup Quaker Oats
- ¼ cup low-fat milk
- ⅓ cup low-fat plain yogurt
- ⅛ teaspoon almond extract
- ½ cup diced mango
- 1 teaspoon honey
- 1 teaspoon chia seeds

Directions

1. Add oats to your container of choice. Pour in low-fat milk and yogurt.
2. Mix in almond extract. Add a layer of mango. Top off with a drizzle of honey and chia seeds.
3. Place in the refrigerator for 3 hours to overnight.

3. Mini Red Velvet Cupcakes with Cream Cheese Icing

Prep Time: 25 mins

Total Time: 1 hr

Servings: 30

Ingredients

Cupcakes:

- 2 ½ cups sifted all-purpose flour
- 1 ½ cups white sugar
- 1 teaspoon salt
- 1 teaspoon baking soda
- 1 teaspoon unsweetened cocoa powder
- 1 ½ cups vegetable oil
- 1 cup buttermilk
- 2 large eggs
- 2 tablespoons red food coloring
- 1 teaspoon vanilla extract
- 1 teaspoon white vinegar

Cream Cheese Icing:

- 3 (6 ounce) packages cream cheese, at room temperature
- 1 cup unsalted butter, at room temperature
- 3 cups sifted confectioners' sugar
- 1 teaspoon vanilla extract

Directions

1. Preheat the oven to 350 degrees F (175 degrees C). Grease 30 mini muffin cups.
2. Sift flour, sugar, salt, baking soda, and cocoa powder together in a bowl.
3. Beat oil, buttermilk, eggs, food coloring, vanilla extract, and vinegar together in the bowl of a stand mixer fitted with the paddle attachment. Slowly add the flour mixture; beat on low speed until batter is just moistened and still airy. Pour batter into the muffin cups.
4. Bake in the preheated oven until a toothpick inserted into the center of a cupcake comes out clean, about 15 minutes. Cool on a wire rack for 5 minutes. Run a table knife around the edges to

loosen. Invert cupcakes carefully onto a serving plate or cooling rack. Let cool, about 15 minutes.

5. Beat cream cheese and butter together in a clean stand mixer bowl. Slowly add confectioners' sugar and vanilla extract. Mix on low until smooth. Spread icing over cooled cupcakes.

4. Amazing Blueberry Rhubarb Pie

Prep Time: 15 mins

Total Time: 3 hrs

Servings: 8

Ingredients

- ¼ cup white sugar
- ¼ cup light brown sugar
- ¼ cup quick-cooking tapioca
- ¼ teaspoon salt
- 3 cups diced rhubarb
- 3 cups fresh blueberries
- 1 pastry for a 9-inch double crust pie

Directions

1. Preheat oven to 400 degrees F (200 degrees C).
2. Stir white sugar, brown sugar, tapioca, and salt together in a large bowl. Add rhubarb and blueberries; toss to coat.
3. Divide the pie dough in half and roll each half out into a 9-inch round. Place 1 round of dough in the

bottom of a pie plate. Pile rhubarb-blueberry mixture on top of the dough and top with the remaining dough round. Trim excess dough from the top crust to leave a 1/2-inch border below the top rim of the pie plate. Tuck the top edges of the crust under the bottom crust and crimp border together. Place pie plate on a rimmed baking sheet.

4. Bake in the preheated oven for 20 minutes. Reduce oven temperature to 350 degrees F (175 degrees C) and continue baking until the crust is golden brown and the filling is bubbling, 25 to 30 minutes more. Cool for 2 hours.

5. Peanut Butter/Chocolate Chip Cookie Bars

Servings: 20

Ingredients

- ½ cup butter
- 1 ½ cups graham cracker crumbs
- 1 (14 ounce) can sweetened condensed milk
- 2 cups semisweet chocolate chips
- 1 cup peanut butter chips

Directions

1. Preheat oven to 350 degrees F.
2. Melt butter over low heat.
3. Pour butter into 13 x 9 inch pan. Sprinkle graham cracker crumbs over butter.
4. Pour condensed milk over crumbs. Sprinkle chocolate and peanut butter chips over milk mixture and press down firmly.
5. Bake 25 to 30 minutes.

Servings: 24

Ingredients

- 1 cup tomato juice
- 1 cup water
- 1 (.25 ounce) package instant yeast
- ¼ cup vegetable oil
- ⅓ cup honey
- ¼ cup chopped fresh parsley
- ¼ cup chopped green onions
- 2 cloves garlic
- 1 carrot, shredded
- 1 teaspoon salt
- 6 cups bread flour

Directions

1. In a sauce pan, heat the tomato juice and water over a low heat until warm to the touch. Pour into a large warmed bowl, and add yeast and honey; stir to dissolve yeast. Allow to rest until yeast is creamy.

2. Mix in oil, parsley, onion, garlic, carrot, and salt. Add 1 cup of the flour, and stir until smooth. Add more flour, until a firm dough is formed. Knead five minutes on a lightly floured surface. Place dough in a greased bowl, and turn to coat the surface completely. Allow to rise in a warm place until doubled in size.

3. Punch down, and divide into halves. Form two loaves, and put into greased 9 x 5 inch loaf pans. Allow to rise for another 45 minutes, or until loaves have doubled in size.

4. Bake at 400 degrees F (220 degrees C) for about 30 minutes, until golden brown. Remove from pans to wire rack to cool.

7. Ham and Pineapple Couscous Salad

Prep Time: 20 mins

Total Time: 25 mins

Servings: 4

Ingredients

- 1 cup water
- 2 tablespoons butter
- ½ teaspoon garlic powder
- 1 cup couscous
- 4 ounces cooked ham, cut into 1/2 inch pieces
- 1 (8 ounce) can pineapple chunks, juice reserved
- ½ small red onion, sliced
- 1 cup frozen green peas, thawed
- 1 tablespoon lemon juice
- Dijon-style prepared mustard
- 1 tablespoon vegetable oil

Directions

1. In a large saucepan, bring water, butter and garlic powder to a boil. Turn off heat and stir in

couscous. Cover and let stand for 5 minutes. Fluff with a fork and let cool.

2. In a large bowl, mix together couscous, ham, pineapple, onion and drained peas

3. In a small bowl whisk together 1/4 cup reserved pineapple juice, lemon juice, Dijon-style mustard and vegetable oil. Pour dressing over the salad and stir to coat. Salt and pepper to taste.

8. Carrot Crust Broccoli Quiche

Prep Time: 15 mins

Total Time: 1 hr 40 mins

Servings: 6

Ingredients

Crust:

- 3 cups shredded carrots
- ¼ cup canola oil
- ¼ cup diced onion
- 1 teaspoon salt substitute
- 1 teaspoon ground black pepper
- ¼ cup cold water
- 2 tablespoons cornstarch

Filling:

- 2 small heads broccoli, shredded
- 3 eggs
- ½ cup pesto sauce
- 1 teaspoon salt substitute

Topping:

- ¼ cup grated Parmesan cheese, or to taste

Directions

1. Preheat oven to 450 degrees F (230 degrees C).
2. Blend carrots, canola oil, onion, 1 teaspoon salt substitute, and pepper together in a blender until smooth. Whisk water and cornstarch together in a bowl until cornstarch is dissolved; add to carrot mixture and blend until smooth. Pour carrot mixture into a 1 1/2-quart casserole dish and press into a 'crust' shape.
3. Bake in the preheated oven until crust is dry and firm, about 20 minutes.
4. Whisk broccoli, eggs, pesto, and 1 teaspoon salt substitute together in a bowl until smooth; pour over the carrot crust.
5. Bake in the preheated oven until set in the middle, 40 to 45 minutes. Cool quiche for 25 minutes and top with Parmesan cheese.

10. Tortas

Prep Time: 20 mins

Total Time: 30 mins

Servings: 4

Ingredients

- 4 (3 ounce) thin-cut beef round steaks
- 4 Mexican-style sandwich rolls (bolillos)
- ¼ cup sour cream, divided
- 1 (15 ounce) can pinto beans - drained, rinsed, and mashed - divided
- 2 avocados - peeled, pitted and sliced
- 2 large tomatoes, sliced
- 2 pickled jalapeno peppers, sliced into quarters lengthwise
- 2 cups shredded romaine lettuce, divided
- 1 cup chopped fresh cilantro, divided
- 1 cup crumbled queso fresco (Mexican fresh cheese), divided
- 1 lime, quartered

Directions

1. Heat a large skillet over medium heat, and pan-
   fry the round steaks 5 minutes on each side, or to
   desired doneness.

2. Slice the rolls lengthwise. Spread about 1
   tablespoon of sour cream onto one side of each
   roll, and top with about 1/3 cup of mashed pinto
   beans per sandwich. Place a cooked round steak
   per sandwich on top of the pinto beans, and then
   layer each sandwich with one-fourth of the
   avocado slices, tomato slices, and sliced pickled
   jalapenos, about 1/2 cup of shredded lettuce, 1/4
   cup of cilantro, and 1/4 cup of crumbled queso
   fresco cheese. Squeeze a lime wedge over each
   sandwich, close, and serve.

11. Peanutty Green Beans

Prep Time: 10 mins

Total Time: 20 mins

Servings: 2

Ingredients

- ⅓ pound trimmed fresh green beans
- 5 tablespoons smooth peanut butter
- 1 teaspoon brown sugar
- ½ teaspoon soy sauce
- ⅓ cup chopped peanuts
- 1 teaspoon miso paste

Directions

1. Bring a large pot of lightly salted water to a boil. Add the green beans and cook uncovered until tender, about 3 minutes. Drain in a colander and immediately immerse in ice water for several minutes until cold to stop the cooking process. Once the green beans are cold, drain well and cut into 2-inch pieces.

2. While the green beans are cooking, stir together the peanut butter, sugar, soy sauce, peanuts, and miso paste in a mixing bowl.

3. Once the green beans have been cut, stir into the peanut sauce and serve.

12. Oven-Roasted Brussels Sprouts with Garlic

Prep Time: 10 mins

Total Time: 25 mins

Servings: 4

Ingredients

- 6 tablespoons olive oil
- 1 pound Brussels sprouts, trimmed and halved lengthwise
- 6 cloves garlic, minced
- salt and ground black pepper to taste
- 1 tablespoon balsamic vinegar

Directions

1. Preheat the oven to 400 degrees F (200 degrees C).
2. Heat oil in a cast iron skillet until shimmering. Place Brussels sprouts carefully in the hot oil, cut-side down. Sprinkle in garlic, salt, and pepper. Cook until Brussels sprouts begin to brown, 3 to 5 minutes.

3. Transfer skillet to the preheated oven and cook until Brussels sprouts are very browned and tender, 10 to 20 minutes. Shake skillet every 5 minutes to ensure even cooking.

4. Season with salt and pepper, stir in balsamic vinegar, and serve immediately.

13. Best Peach Cobbler Ever

Prep Time: 30 mins

Total Time: 1 hr 30 mins

Servings: 18

Ingredients

- 1 (29 ounce) can sliced peaches
- 2 tablespoons butter, melted
- 1 pinch ground cinnamon
- 1 pinch ground nutmeg
- 1 tablespoon cornstarch
- ½ cup water
- 1 cup milk
- 1 cup white sugar
- 1 cup all-purpose flour
- 2 teaspoons baking powder
- 1 pinch salt
- ½ cup butter
- 1 teaspoon ground cinnamon
- ¼ teaspoon ground nutmeg

Directions

1. Preheat oven to 350 degrees F (175 degrees C.) In a large bowl, combine sliced peaches with juice, 2 tablespoons melted butter, a pinch of cinnamon and a pinch of nutmeg. Dissolve cornstarch in water, then stir into peach mixture; set aside.

2. In another bowl, combine milk, sugar, flour, baking powder and salt. Beat until smooth - mixture will be thin.

3. Melt 1/2 cup butter in a 9x13 inch pan. Pour batter over melted butter. Spoon peaches over batter. Sprinkle top with additional cinnamon and nutmeg.

4. Bake in preheated oven for 1 hour, or until knife inserted comes out clean.

Servings: 24

Ingredients

- 1 cup semisweet chocolate chips
- ½ cup rum
- ¼ cup light corn syrup
- 3 cups vanilla wafer crumbs
- 1 ½ cups chopped pecans
- 1 cup confectioners' sugar
- 24 red candied cherries, halved

Directions

1. Melt the chocolate chips and stir in the rum and corn syrup.
2. Stir together the vanilla wafer crumbs, pecans and 1/2 cup of the confectioners' sugar. Drizzle the chocolate mixture over the crumb mixture and stir until blended.
3. Shape mixture into 1 inch balls. Roll balls in the remaining confectioners' sugar. Place cherry half in center of each cookie, pressing down lightly.

Store in an airtight container for several days to develop flavor.

Prep Time: 15 mins

Total Time: 40 mins

Servings: 4

Ingredients

- 4 baking potatoes, peeled and cubed
- 2 skinless, boneless chicken breast halves - diced
- 2 medium red bell peppers, chopped
- 1 large white onion, chopped
- 3 celery ribs, chopped
- 2 cups favorite barbeque sauce

Directions

1. Make four foil packets by the following method, using 1-foot squares of heavy duty aluminum foil: fold square in half and smooth flat. Seal each of the narrow ends by folding over each edge three times to make a 1/4-inch border, smoothing flat after every fold. You should now have a foil packet that is open on one long side. Repeat to form four packets.

2. In a bowl or resealable plastic bag, combine the potatoes, chicken cubes, red peppers, onion, celery, and barbeque sauce; mix well. Evenly divide the mixture among the foil packets. Roll up the open end of the packets to seal.

3. Place packets on a grill over the coals of a fire. Cook until the potatoes are tender and the chicken is fully cooked, about 25 minutes, depending on the intensity of the heat.

16. No Bake Bumpy Peanut Butter Nuggets

Prep Time: 15 mins

Total Time: 1 hr 15 mins

Servings: 30

Ingredients

- ½ cup natural peanut butter
- ¼ cup nonfat dry milk powder
- ¼ cup unsweetened flaked coconut
- ⅓ cup rolled oats
- ½ teaspoon ground cinnamon
- ¼ cup wheat germ
- ¼ cup unsweetened apple juice concentrate, thawed

Directions

1. Combine peanut butter, milk powder, and coconut in a large mixing bowl. Stir in oats, ground cinnamon, wheat germ, and apple juice concentrate until thoroughly combined.

water. Carefully open up the caul fat on a clean work surface, and cut into 4 inch (10 cm) squares.

3. Place a small compressed handful of the sausage near the edge of one square. Fold the sides over, and roll up firmly. Repeat with remaining meat and fat until you have about 10 sausages.

4. Prepare a charcoal grill for high heat. Place sausages onto skewers.

5. Grill the sausages for 20 minutes, turning frequently until the outside is crispy and dark, and the inside is no longer pink.

18. Our Favorite Most Amazing Guacamole

Prep Time: 10 mins

Total Time: 10 mins

Servings: 4

Ingredients

- 3 each ripe avocados - halved, pitted, and peeled
- 1 lime
- 10 each cherry tomatoes, or to taste
- 1 shallot, minced
- 2 tablespoons chopped fresh cilantro, or to taste
- 1 clove garlic, minced, or to taste
- ¼ teaspoon kosher salt, or to taste
- 1 pinch ground multi-colored peppercorns, or to taste

Directions

1. Place avocados in a medium bowl and squeeze in lime juice. Add tomatoes, shallot, cilantro, garlic, salt, and pepper. Mash with an immersion blender or a sturdy fork until avocado is mashed

and ingredients are combined. Stir gently and
serve immediately.

19. Secret Ingredient Smoothie

Prep Time: 10 mins

Total Time: 10 mins

Servings: 1

Ingredients

- 3 cups chopped romaine lettuce
- ⅓ cup milk, or more as needed
- 4 frozen strawberries, or more to taste
- 1 frozen banana, cut into chunks
- ¼ teaspoon vanilla extract, or to taste

Directions

1. Put romaine lettuce into the bottom of a blender pitcher; add enough milk to cover completely and blend on High until smooth.
2. Drop one strawberry at a time into the blender while still running on High and allow the berry to blend completely before adding the next. Blend one banana chunk at a time into the mixture in the same manner as the strawberries. Thin the smoothie with additional milk to keep smoothie

blending properly. Blend vanilla extract into the smoothie.

Servings: 10

Ingredients

- ⅔ cup butter
- ¼ cup Dijon-style prepared mustard
- 1 ¼ cups dried bread crumbs, seasoned
- ¼ cup Parmesan cheese
- 20 chicken wings, tips discarded

Directions

1. Preheat oven to 400 degrees F (205 degrees C).
2. Melt butter or margarine and stir in mustard. Place bread crumbs in a flat dish. Roll each chicken piece in the butter mixture, then coat with bread crumbs.
3. Place chicken pieces in a 9x13 inch baking dish. Sprinkle with cheese and bake in the preheated oven for 15 minutes. Turn and bake 15 minutes longer, or until crispy.

Servings: 12

Ingredients

- 1 cup cornmeal
- ½ cup milk
- ½ cup shortening
- ½ cup white sugar
- 1 ⅓ cups cake flour
- 2 ½ teaspoons baking powder
- 1 teaspoon salt
- 1 egg
- 1 cup milk

Directions

1. Preheat oven to 350 degrees F (175 degrees C). Grease thoroughly an 8 inch square cake pan.
2. Combine cornmeal and milk. Sift flour, baking powder, and salt. Stir together the egg and milk.
3. Cream shortening, and blend in sugar. Stir flour mixture and egg mixture alternately into creamed mixture alternately. Blend in cornmeal mixture.

4. Bake for 40 to 45 minutes. Serve hot, with maple syrup.

Prep Time: 5 mins

Total Time: 50 mins

Servings: 5

Ingredients

- 5 large Granny Smith apples
- wooden craft sticks
- 1 (14 ounce) package individually wrapped caramels, unwrapped
- 2 tablespoons water
- 7 ounces chocolate candy bar, broken into pieces
- 2 tablespoons shortening, divided
- 1 cup colored candy coating melts

Directions

1. Bring a large pot of water to a boil. Dip apples into boiling water briefly, using a slotted spoon, to remove any wax that may be present. Wipe dry, and set aside to cool. Insert sticks into the apples through the cores.

2. Line a baking sheet with waxed paper and coat with cooking spray. Place the unwrapped caramels into a microwave-safe medium bowl along with 2 tablespoons of water. Cook on high for 2 minutes, then stir and continue cooking and stirring at 1 minute intervals until caramel is melted and smooth.

3. Hold apples by the stick, and dip into the caramel to coat. Set on waxed paper; refrigerate for about 15 minutes to set.

4. Heat the chocolate with 1 tablespoon of shortening in a microwave-safe bowl until melted and smooth. Dip apples into the chocolate to cover the layer of caramel. Return to the waxed paper to set.

5. Melt the candy melts in the microwave with the remaining shortening, stirring every 30 seconds until smooth. Use a fork or wooden stick to flick colored designs onto your apples for a finishing touch. Refrigerate until set, overnight is even better.

23. Raspberry Napoleons Dessert

Prep Time: 15 mins

Total Time: 35 mins

Servings: 16

Ingredients

- 1 (17.5 ounce) package frozen puff pastry, thawed
- 1 (8 ounce) package cream cheese, softened
- ½ cup white sugar
- 2 tablespoons 35% heavy whipping cream
- 1 teaspoon lemon zest
- 1 pint fresh raspberries
- 3 tablespoons confectioners' sugar, or as needed

Directions

1. Preheat oven to 350 degrees F (175 degrees C). Line 2 baking sheets with parchment paper.
2. Roll out 1 puff pastry sheet on a floured work surface until it is 1/4-inch thick. Cut into 16 squares. Transfer to a baking sheet and prick all

over with a fork. Repeat with remaining puff pastry sheet.

3. Bake in the preheated oven until lightly browned on the top and bottom, 10 to 15 minutes. Let cool, about 10 minutes.

4. Combine cream cheese, white sugar, heavy cream, and lemon zest in a bowl. Mix by hand until smooth and glossy. Dollop cream cheese mixture over 16 squares. Spread out cream cheese mixture and cover with raspberries. Top with the remaining puff pastry squares and dust with confectioners' sugar.

Prep Time: 25 mins

Total Time: 40 mins

Servings: 2

Ingredients

- 1 large tomato, diced
- 2 tablespoons chopped red onion
- ½ cup chopped cilantro
- ½ teaspoon honey
- 1 teaspoon lime juice
- 1 tablespoon balsamic vinegar
- Salt and pepper to taste
- 1 tablespoon bacon grease
- 1 clove garlic, minced
- 2 tablespoons minced red onion
- 1 (15.5 ounce) can black beans, drained and rinsed
- 2 tablespoons water

Directions

1. Stir together the tomato, onion, cilantro, and honey. Season with lime juice, vinegar, salt and pepper; set aside.

2. Melt bacon grease in a saucepan over medium heat. Stir in garlic and onion, cook until softened and translucent, about 3 minutes. Pour in the black beans and water, season to taste with salt and pepper, then simmer for 10 minutes or until hot. Serve topped with pico de gallo.

25. Kool-Aid Popcorn

Prep Time: 10 mins

Total Time: 45 mins

Servings: 20

Ingredients

- 6 quarts popped popcorn
- 2 cups white sugar
- 1 cup light corn syrup
- ⅔ cup butter
- 2 (.13 ounce) envelopes unsweetened soft drink mix, any flavor
- 1 teaspoon baking soda

Directions

1. Preheat oven to 225 degrees F (110 degrees C). Grease a large baking sheet. Place popped popcorn in a large bowl.
2. Combine sugar, corn syrup, and butter in a saucepan; bring to a boil until sugar dissolves, about 3 minutes.

3. Combine drink mix and baking soda in a large bowl; pour sugar mixture into drink mixture, stirring carefully. Sugar mixture will bubble. Pour mixture over popcorn; toss to evenly coat. Transfer coated popcorn to baking sheet.

4. Bake in the preheated oven, stirring every 10 minutes, until coating has hardened, about 30 minutes. Cool and break popcorn into pieces.

26. Easy Pineapple Sorbet

Prep Time: 5 mins

Total Time: 5 hrs 5 mins

Servings: 6

Ingredients

- 1 ½ cups orange juice
- 1 cup frozen pineapple chunks

Directions

1. Mix orange juice and pineapple in a blender on high speed until smooth. Transfer to a covered container; freeze for at least 5 hours.

Prep Time: 15 mins

Total Time: 4 hrs 35 mins

Servings: 32

Ingredients

- 2 ½ pounds fresh peaches - peeled, pitted and chopped
- 1 pint half-and-half cream
- ½ cup white sugar
- 1 (14 ounce) can sweetened condensed milk
- 1 (12 fluid ounce) can evaporated milk
- 1 teaspoon vanilla extract
- 2 cups whole milk, or as needed

Directions

1. Working in batches, purée peaches with half-and-half and sugar in a blender or food processor.
2. Mix together peach mixture, sweetened condensed milk, evaporated milk, and vanilla in a gallon ice cream freezer container. Pour enough

whole milk into the container to reach the fill line, about 2 cups.

3. Pour mixture into an ice cream maker and freeze according to manufacturer's instructions, about 20 minutes. Transfer to an airtight container and freeze until firm, about 4 hours.

Prep Time: 15 mins

Total Time: 3 hrs 50 mins

Servings: 10

Ingredients

- ¼ cup pineapple juice
- ¼ cup coconut oil
- 1 ½ teaspoons vanilla extract
- ½ teaspoon ground cinnamon
- ½ teaspoon sea salt
- 3 cups rolled oats
- ¼ cup sunflower seeds
- ½ cup pitted dates
- ¼ cup roasted almonds
- 1 ¼ cups quick-cooking oats
- ½ cup raisins
- ½ cup dried cranberries

Directions

1. Preheat the oven to 200 degrees F (95 degrees C). Lightly grease a baking sheet.

2. Mix pineapple juice and coconut oil together in a microwave-safe bowl or jar and melt in a microwave, about 1 minute. Add vanilla extract, cinnamon, and salt; stir.

3. Pour rolled oats and sunflower seeds into a large bowl.

4. Place dates and almonds into an electric blender with pineapple juice mixture. Pulse for about 15 seconds to combine. Pour into oat mixture and stir using a large spoon. Stir in quick-cooking oats. Pour onto the prepared baking sheet evenly.

5. Bake in the preheated oven for 2 1/2 hours. Remove from the oven and add raisins and cranberries. Continue to bake until golden, about 30 minutes more. Let cool for 30 minutes before serving.

Servings: 12

Ingredients

- ⅓ cup boiling water
- 2 cups dates, pitted and chopped
- ½ cup shortening
- 1 cup white sugar
- ⅛ teaspoon ground cinnamon
- ¾ teaspoon salt
- ⅛ teaspoon ground nutmeg
- 2 eggs
- 1 cup all-purpose flour
- ¼ teaspoon baking soda
- ½ cup chopped walnuts
- ¼ cup confectioners' sugar

Directions

1. In a small bowl, pour boiling water over dates, and set aside to cool. Preheat oven to 325 degrees F (165 degrees C). Grease a 10x10 inch baking pan.

2. In a medium bowl, cream together the shortening
   and white sugar. Add eggs, one at a time, beating
   after each addition. Add the dates, including any
   water; mix well. Sift together the flour, cinnamon,
   salt, nutmeg, and baking soda; stir into the date
   mixture. Then stir in the nuts.

3. Spread the mixture evenly into the prepared
   10x10 inch pan, and bake for 45 minutes in the
   preheated oven. When cool, cut into bars, and roll
   each bar in confectioners' sugar.

30. Spooky Halloween Chili

Prep Time: 10 mins

Total Time: 6 hrs 10 mins

Servings: 8

Ingredients

- ½ pound ground beef
- 2 (16 ounce) cans chili beans
- 1 (14.5 ounce) can stewed tomatoes
- ½ (10 ounce) package frozen corn
- 3 tablespoons apple cider
- 1 tablespoon chili powder

Directions

1. Mix ground beef, chili beans, stewed tomatoes, corn, apple cider, and chili powder in a large pot over high heat; bring to a simmer, reduce heat to medium-low, and cook until the beef is cooked and tender, about 6 hours.

www.ingramcontent.com/pod-product-compliance
Lightning Source LLC
Chambersburg PA
CBHW070727260726
48660CB00007B/2764